Dr. Michael

GW00673155

PERFECT POSTURE

The Basis of Power

*The prime secret for performance
that every athlete and regular
exerciser needs to know.*

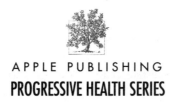

APPLE PUBLISHING
PROGRESSIVE HEALTH SERIES

The Information contained in this book was prepared from medical and scientific sources which are referenced herein and are believed to be accurate and reliable. However, the opinions expressed herein by the author do not necessarily represent the opinions or the views of the publisher. Nor should the information herein be used to treat or to prevent any medical condition unless it is used with the full knowledge, compliance and agreement of our personal physician or other licensed health care professional. Readers are strongly advised to seek the advice of their personal health care professional(s) before proceeding with any changes in any health care program.

National Library of Canada Cataloguing in Publication

Colgan, Michael
    Perfect posture : the basis of power : the prime secret for performance that every athlete and regular exerciser needs to know / Michael Colgan.

(Progressive health series)
Includes bibliographical references.
ISBN 1-896817-24-6

    1. Posture. 2. Stretching exercises. I. Title. II. Series.

RA781.5.C64 2002　　　　　　　**613.7'8**　　　　　**C2002-901277-5**

Apple Publishing Company Ltd.
220 East 59th Avenue
Vancouver, British Columbia
Canada V5X 1X9 Tel: (604) 214-6688   Fax: (604) 214-3566

E-mail: books@applepublishing.com　　　**Website: www.applepublishing.com**

10　　*9*　　*8*　　*7*　　*6*　　*5*　　*4*　　*3*　　*2*　　*1*

CONTENTS

Perfect Posture 5

Cultural Demands 6

Longevity 7

Ideal Posture 7

Spinal Curves 11

Spinal Flexibility 13

Maintaining Spinal Flexibility 16

Spine: Anterior View 17

Spine: Posterior View 18

Testing and Correction of Muscle Imbalance 20

Rotator Cuff 21

Pectorals 23

Pectoralis Minor 24

Pectoralis Major 24

Teres, Rhomboids, and Latissimus 25

Hip Flexors 26

Stretching Hip Flexors 28

Tensor Fascia Lata 29

Hamstrings 30

Muscles of the Core 32

Testing Abdominal Strength 33

Prescription for a Top Trainer 35

Form 1 For Postural and Structural Analysis 37

Form 2 For Postural and Structural Analysis 38

Form 3 For Postural and Structural Analysis 39

References 40

PERFECT POSTURE

The soaring incidence of postural defects in Western Society stems from three main sources: domestication, cultural demands, and longevity. Over the last 100 years, domestication of the human species has accelerated faster than at any other time in history. Our labour-saving culture has eliminated almost all need and motivation for folk to exert themselves. Less than 20% of American adults do any regular exercise.[1-4]

We have become cosseted "battery humans" that move of our own volition little more than the battery chickens we eat. We impose this sedentary lifestyle on a superb anatomical structure that developed in concert with our violent evolution, and requires similar vigorous activity to maintain it.[1] Our current chronic rate of disuse destroys bone, muscle, and connective tissue alike.[5,6]

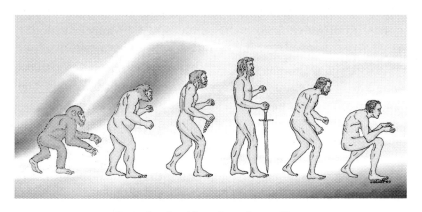

Figure 1. Effects of modern life on the evolution of human structure.

CULTURAL DEMANDS

The second major cause of structural defects is a cosmic irony. When our primate ancestors stood up and released their front paws, to evolve the unique hands and manual dexterity that enabled us to develop complex communication and become human, they also put a kink in the spine. Over millions of years, their hip flexors stretched, their hamstrings stretched, and the muscles and connective tissues of the back thickened and shortened, to hold up the spine and change its shape, and straighten the legs against gravity. Thus, humans became the only creatures capable of true upright posture.[7]

But the very manual dexterity that encouraged human intelligence to evolve, is now pressed into service by cultural demands, almost from birth, to compel us to show written evidence of mental competence. We spend 10 -15 years bent over desks, work tables and computers learning to read, write and cipher, and to precisely manipulate small objects. Most of us then spend another 40 years or so earning a living in largely the same manner.

This habitual seated crouch shortens the hip flexors and hamstrings and overstretches the back muscles and connective tissues, all of which distorts the human spine.[8,9] Many of us today spend most of our lives in pre-human postures unsuited to our physiological evolution, and thereby develop numerous defects and weaknesses. Look around your local pub or coffee bar. The average posture resembles that of a consumptive chimpanzee.

LONGEVITY

The third cause of postural defects is our newfound longevity. From an abbreviated lifespan of 53 a century ago, we continue to shuffle on today to a ripe old 77.[10] That span gives gravity a great deal more time before death to pull down the structure. You see double chins everywhere, but you never see a double forehead.

"Time to kill" provides an apt description of Western Society. And our pandering, paper-mad, milksop culture is hellbent on selling the damaging lifestyle, which ensures that the killing occurs.

IDEAL POSTURE

Riding the medical knowledge explosion of the Internet, the multitude of aging and ailing baby boomers, are making the tardy discovery that their bodies need not degenerate as quickly as those of their parents. And hordes of them flock to the gyms, and hire personal trainers galore, to bully reluctant bodies back into youthful shape. But, to their consternation, imposing such bully-begotten strength on a defective structure only ages and ails them more.

Unless you first analyse the structure, and design corrective measures as an integral part of every resistance exercise program, the hard-won muscle will only increase defects and distortions, and will hasten, rather than reverse, degeneration.

The recent realisation of the importance of sound structure has authorities fighting like banshees over what constitutes ideal posture. Figure 2 shows the side view of the Colgan Institute model. By no means the final word, it represents a compromise between some of the more sensible texts,[11,12] and our measurements of thousands of athletes over the last 27 years.

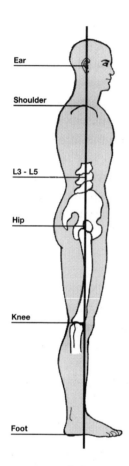

Figure 2. Ideal Posture

The plumbline divides the body into two halves of approximately equal weight. The six main landmarks are: the ear, the shoulder, lumbar vertebrae L3-L5, the hip, the knee, and the foot.

Ear

The plumb line passes just behind the meatus (passage) of the ear. In subjects with good posture it usually falls through the rear of the ear lobe. But ears differ widely in shape and position, and the line may fall behind the lobe.

Shoulder

The plumb line falls through the midline of the normal shoulder joint. One common postural defect that displaces the shoulder landmark is a winged scapula. If the scapula is not flat on the back, the shoulder joint moves forward, out of the balanced position, and the line falls behind it. The opposite problem occurs in athletes with large shoulder and triceps development. The line appears to fall in front of the midline, although the joint may be in ideal position.

Lumbar Vertebrae L3-L5

The plumbline falls through the midline of lumbar vertebrae L3-L5. You can observe this landmark only in slim subjects dressed in minimal sportswear. It helps analysis if you locate the rear of the vertebrae manually.

Hip

The plumbline falls just behind the axis of the hip. You can identify this landmark by getting the subject to flex the hip and place a finger on the axis of rotation. The most common postural defect that displaces the hip landmark is forward tilting of the pelvis. Ideally the pelvis should be level, such that the anterior superior spines are in vertical line with the front of the symphysis pubis (junction of the pubic bones). This position enables the front-to-back stabilizing muscles to have equal lines of pull. For example, the rectus femoris of the quadriceps, the tensor fascia lata and the sartorius, all pull down from their attachments on the anterior iliac spines, while the obliques and the rectus abdominus pull up from their attachments on or near the pubic bones.

More than 60% of adult Americans over 40 have lost oblique and rectus abdominus support. Women often lose this function because of childbirth which is not followed by essential rehabilitation exercises for the abdomen. Men mostly lose the function because of disuse. The result is forward tilting of the pelvis, which increases the lumbar curve, causing low back pain and excessive wearing stress on the lumbar spine.

The angle between the pelvis and the thigh also decreases, putting the hip habitually in partial flexion, which quickly exhausts the hip flexors in any standing, bending, walking or running movements. Any leg exercise routine, which does not also include a comprehensive remedial program for this condition, will only make it worse, and will cause severe degeneration of the lumbar spine in later life.[14]

Knee

The plumbline falls just in front of the axis of the knee joint. In numerous exercise and gym texts, however, you will see diagrams showing the plumb line passing through the centre of both hip and knee joints. Such diagrams demonstrate an understanding of human anatomy somewhat less than that of the average bear.

The vertical positioning of the hip and knee joint follows a locking principle well known in engineering. The axis of the knee joint is designed to be behind the plumb line, and the axis of the hip joint in front of the plumbline, thereby stabilizing both joints in extension. This design requires the least muscular effort to prevent flexion, and allows the bone shapes, tendons and ligaments to passively resist hyperextension. To maintain this important stability chain, the Colgan Power Program does not use exercises that hyperextend the hip or hyperflex the knee, or that unnecessarily stretch the hamstrings.

Loss of hip/knee stability is especially obvious in the "old man" posture of partially flexed knees and hips, which makes standing, walking and running exhausting and uncomfortable activities, because the hip, thigh, knee and lower leg muscles are constantly overworking against gravity to prevent flexion and keep the body upright.

Foot

The plumb line falls in front of the outer malleolus of the ankle and approximately through the centre of the arch of the foot.

SPINAL CURVES

Once you have established the plumb line for an individual, the next step is to measure the spinal curves. The spine has a fixed sacral curve at the buttocks, and three flexible curves, lumbar at the lower back, thoracic at the upper back, and cervical at the neck.

In attempts to simplify this complicated design, some texts suggest that ideal posture occurs only when all three flexible curves are approximately equal, and at 35° apiece. Because of individual differences in anatomy and muscle attachment, however, spinal curves in ideal posture show a considerable range of variation. The curves are rarely equal and vary widely from 35°.

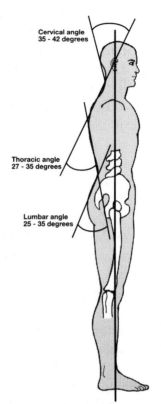

Figure 3. Spinal Curves

From the work of the most respected authorities,[12,13] and from our own measurements at the Colgan Institute, in ideal posture the cervical curve is usually largest, and varies from 33-42° (in deviation from the vertical and return to the vertical). As illustrated in Figure 3, the thoracic curve varies from 27-35°, and the lumbar curve from 25-35°. Only outside these ranges can you reasonably judge either insufficient or excessive spinal curvature.

The most common defects are :

1. Excessive cervical curve, caused primarily by habitual forward head carriage.

2. Excessive thoracic curve, caused primarily by slumping of shoulders from habitual bad posture, or from over-development of the muscles of the front of the torso.

3. Excessive lumbar curve, caused primarily by collapse of the lower abdominal wall, shortening of the hip flexors, and anterior tilting of the pelvis.

Examine the amazing complexity of the normal spine illustrated in Figure 4. Every vertebra is different. Everything fits together exactly,

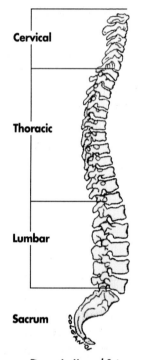

Figure 4. Normal Spine

better than the finest of jigsaw puzzles. If even one space between the vertebrae is compressed, or if even one vertebra is being pulled out of place, then the spine is compromised and optimal function is impossible. Imposing a resistance exercise program on a defective spine will only worsen the problem. Postural analysis is the essential first step in correct design of every resistance exercise program.

SPINAL FLEXIBILITY

It is the flexibility of the spine that allows you to have spring in your step and snap in your movements. Imposing resistance exercise programs on a stiff spine only further restricts movement. You should examine all subjects for spinal flexibility, and recommend remedial stretching where necessary, before starting any resistance exercise program that puts the back under compression.

Spinal Flexion

Normal flexion of the lumbar spine allows the spine to flatten and remove the lumbar curve. Inability to flatten the spine while lying supine, however, may be caused by short hip flexors. Test hip flexors first (detailed ahead), before concluding that the lumbar spine is stiff and needs remedial exercise. Two good remedial exercises from the Colgan Power Program are Moonwalk and Finding Spinal Curve.

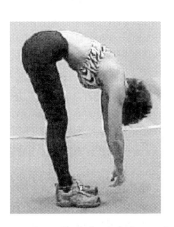
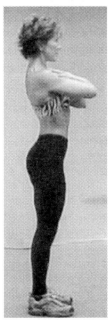
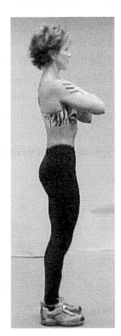

Figure 5. Finding spinal curve. Left to right, flexion, excessive curve, normal curve.

Normal flexion of the thoracic spine is best judged by using the Back Extension Curl-up from the Colgan Power Program shown in Figure 6. This test should show a smooth increase in the posterior curve. The same exercise can be used for remedial work.

Normal flexion of the cervical spine allows the chin to rest on the the sternum at the foot of the neck. Forward neck flexion is seldom a problem, although

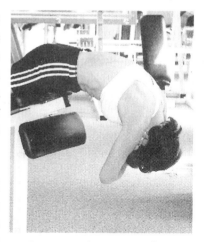

Figure 6. Back Extension Curl-up

overall lack of neck flexibility is common. Exercises for increasing neck flexibility are given in Lee Parore's *Power Posture*.

Lateral flexion of the spine is difficult to measure. The standing side bend often used, combines spinal flexion plus length of the lateral trunk muscles and hip abductors. Useful only as a gross measure, this test suggests normal lateral flexion when the fingertips can reach to below the base of the patella (kneecap).

Spinal Extension

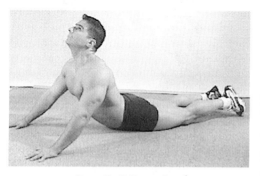

Figure 7. McKenzie Stretch

Some texts use backward bending while standing to measure spinal extension. This measure is of little use, because it combines the three spinal curves in one motion, and also depends on the length of hamstrings and hip flexors. You need something a little more accurate.

To measure extension of the lumbar spine, lie the subject prone (face down) on the table with legs straight and together and feet extended. Apply pressure to the back of the thighs and gastrocnemius. With hands behind head, subject raises torso, keeping anterior superior iliac spines on table. The angle between the table and a line through the shoulder midline and iliac spine should be 15-25°. A good remedial exercise to correct stiffness is the McKenzie Stretch shown in Figure 7, which somewhat mimics the test procedure.

Normal extension of the thoracic spine is simply the ability to flatten the posterior curve while standing, from its normal 27-35° angle to zero. A good remedial exercise for a stiff thoracic spine is the Back Extension Curl-up in Figure 6.

Normal extension of the cervical spine while standing, allows the front of the neck to assume a vertical line when viewed from the side. Refer to Lee Parore's book *Power Posture* for remedial exercises.

MAINTAINING SPINAL FLEXIBILITY

As Lee Parore shows, every good exercise program should contain elements for spinal flexibility, in order to maintain spring, snap, and coordination of movement.[14] Two exercises from the Colgan Power Program, shown in Figure 8, Lying spinal curve, and Hula, help to achieve this goal.

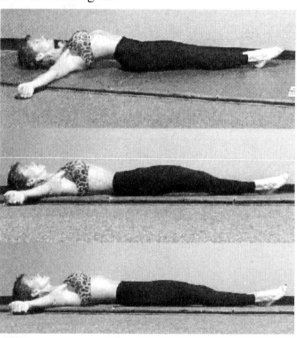

Figure 8. Lying spinal curve.
Top to bottom, excess, flat, normal.

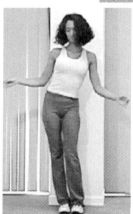

Hula

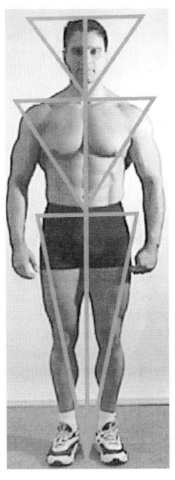

Figure 9. Posture: Anterior View

SPINE: ANTERIOR VIEW

Viewed from the front, the body resembles three inverted pyramids balanced on top of each other. The plumbline divides the body into two equal halves, as shown in Figure 9. The line falls through the center of the head, neck, ribs, groin, and central between the feet. Examine the subject for deviations from the line. Then use a builder's level to determine horizontal balance of shoulders, pelvis and knees.

Head
Observe head carriage and note any irregularity, either in bending of the head to one side, or in deviation of the centre of the head from the plumb line.

Neck
Note any bend of the neck to one side or deviation of the centre of the neck from the plumbline.

Shoulders
Place a level across the bony prominences of the collar bones and note any deviation from the horizontal. Note any deviation of the centre of the chest from the line.

Hips

Place a level across the top of the anterior superior spines of the pelvis and note any deviation from the horizontal. Note any deviation of the belly button from the centerline.

Knees

Place a level across the top of the kneecaps and note any deviation from the horizontal. Note any difference between the distances of the knees from the line.

Feet

The ankle joint is not in a direct front-to-back plane. The anatomy shows that it begins anterior to the medial ankle bone, and ends posterior to the lateral ankle bone. Consequently, oversimplified descriptions of the ideal stance given in some texts, showing feet pointing straight forward, are pure baloney. Human anatomy naturally positions the foot at a 5-15° angle out from the midline. Less than 5° denotes pigeon toes: more than 15° denotes duckfeet. Both require remedial exercises in conjunction with any resistance exercise program. Get the subject to stand correctly before beginning every set of every standing exercise, and to maintain correct foot position throughout the exercise.

Note also any difference between the distances of the feet from the plumbline, and whether the subject stands evenly on each foot, or on the outside or inside edge. Get the subject to stand evenly on the feet for every set of every standing exercise.

SPINE: POSTERIOR VIEW

Viewed from the back, the plumbline divides the body into two equal halves, as shown in Figure 10. The spine is straight, and the head, neck, shoulders, and pelvis central. Examine the subject for deviations from the line. Then use a level to determine horizontal balance of shoulders and pelvis.

Head

Observe head carriage and note any irregularity, either in bending of the head to one side, or in deviation of the centre of the head from the plumbline.

Neck

Note any bend of the neck to one side or deviation of the center of the neck from the plumbline.

Shoulders

Place a level across in line with the bony prominences of the collar

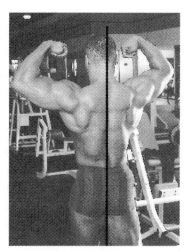

Figure 10. Posture: Posterior view

bones. Note any deviation from the horizontal. Note also any side-to-side deviation of the center of the spine from the line.

Pelvis

Place a level across the body in line with top of bony prominences of the hips. Note any deviation from the horizontal. Note also any side-to-side deviation of the center of the spine from the line.

Scoliosis

Scoliosis denotes a lateral curve of the spine. It is often caused by congenital bone deformity or neuromuscular disease. The most common cause, however, is habitual faulty posture. Habitually lying on the non-dominant side while reading and writing, or habitually carrying a heavy briefcase in the dominant hand, can easily cause scoliosis.

The subject should be examined both standing, and sitting with legs hanging free. Scoliosis present when standing, which disappears when sitting, is often caused by differing leg lengths, and can be corrected by a lift pad in one shoe. Scoliosis which remains present when sitting, is not caused by differing leg lengths, and you should not attempt correction using a shoe lift. You should not use any spinal flexibility exercises either, as these will worsen the condition.

Whatever the cause of scoliosis, muscle imbalances are always present in the trunk, hips, or legs. You can determine these imbalances by testing. Then use exercises to strengthen the weak muscles, and stretches to lengthen the tight muscles. Such remedial exercises will almost always improve the scoliosis when used in conjunction with a good resistance program.

TESTING AND CORRECTION OF MUSCLE IMBALANCE

Common problems of subjects wishing to undertake resistance exercise programs, are forward head posture, forward shoulder carriage, and a lumbar spinal angle exceeding 35°. In most cases the pelvis also shows anterior tilt, with some flexion of the hips. Because these problems involve many of the major muscles of the body, we will use them as examples for testing and correction of muscle length.

Test for shoulder function, short, tight low back erector spinae, tight hip flexors, and tight adductors and abductors. Rectus abdominus and obliques are usually too long and weak. Quadratus lumborum and serratus posterior inferior are often short and tight, restricting spinal rotation and compressing the low back.

Forward head and shoulder carriage and excessive lumbar curve are serious postural faults requiring careful analysis and corrective action. Any resistance program imposed upon them without

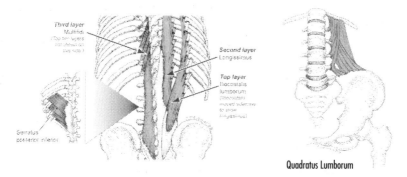

Figure 11. Erector spinae and other major muscles of the lower back that are often tight in athletes.

accompanying remedial action, will only worsen these conditions, by shortening tight muscles even further and increasing stress on the neck, upper back, and lumbar spine. The neck is beyond the scope of this course and is covered in Lee Parore's book *Power Posture*. Here we begin by examining the shoulder.

ROTATOR CUFF

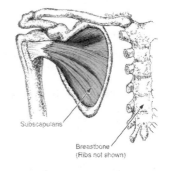

The shoulder is the most mobile joint in the body. To achieve this mobility, the joint does not have a bony socket like the hip, but relies on four small muscles to hold the humerus bone firmly in a shallow depression of flesh. Shown in Figure 12, these muscles of the rotator cuff are the: infraspinatus, supraspinatus, subscapularis, and teres minor.

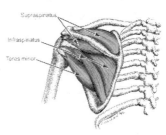

Figure 12. The four muscles of the rotator cuff all originate on the scapula.

All four rotator cuff muscles originate on the scapula and insert on the humerus. Because they are hardly visible, most books on resistance training barely mention them, and offer few if any exercises to strengthen them. Consequently they are sorely neglected in sports training, and are weak in many athletes that we test. In these cases, overbuilt deltoids, pectorals, biceps and triceps, can easily yank the humerus out of position, making rotator cuff injury a frequent upper body problem in athletes.

Testing is easily accomplished using the four internal and external rotation exercises shown in the *New Power Program*. On internal and external rotations from top to bottom, one of which is shown in Figure 13, minimal acceptable strength in men of overall average strength, permits moving a 30lb (14kg) resistance with good form for eight repetitions. Minimal acceptable strength in women of overall average strength, permits moving a 24lb (11kg) resistance for eight repetitions.

On internal and external rotations from bottom to top, minimal acceptable strength in men of overall average strength, permits moving a 24lb (11kg) resistance with good form for eight repetitions. Minimal acceptable strength in women of overall average strength, permits moving an 18lb (8kg) resistance for eight repetitions.

Normal shoulder function includes the ability to raise the arm straight overhead, raise the straight arm diagonally, and to the side, place the bent arms behind the back so that one hand reaching back over the shoulder can tip the fingers of the other hand placed up behind the back. These functions are often compromised, especially in athletes who use bodybuilding exercises, which overbuild and tighten the muscles of the chest and back.

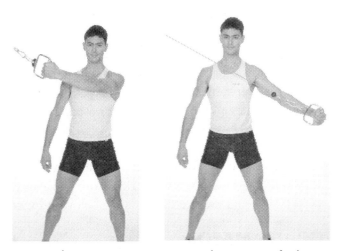

Figure 13. External Rotations Top To Bottom, a strengthening exercise for the rotator cuff.

PECTORALS

Main muscles of the front of the shoulder that give trouble because they are too tight, are the pectoralis minor, overlaid by the pectoralis major.

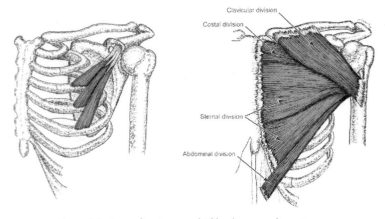

Figure 14. Pectoralis minor overlaid by the pectoralis major.

PECTORALIS MINOR

Test the pectoralis minor first. Subject lies supine (on back), arms straight, elbows down, palms up, knees bent up, low back flat. If shoulders lie flat on table, then length of pectoralis minor is usually normal. If one or both shoulders are raised, then pectoralis minor is short on the raised sides.

Good stretching exercises for a tight pectoralis minor include, upper body stretches Numbers 1 and 3, from the *New Power Program* pp 52-53, and the exercises shown below in Figure 15.

PECTORALIS MAJOR

Subject lies supine, knees bent up, back flat. Abduct straight arm diagonally up with palm supine (palm up). If arm remains flat on table, then the lower and medial fibers of pectoralis major are usually of normal length. If arm hangs up off the table, then pectoralis major is short. Use the same remedial exercises as for pectoralis minor.

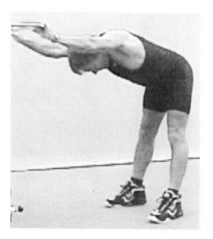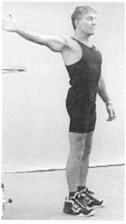

Figure 15. Stretches for tight pectoralis major and minor.

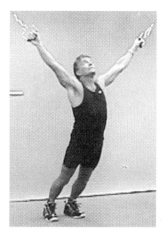 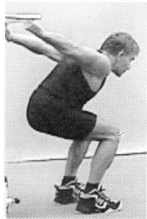

Figure 15. Stretches for tight pectoralis major and minor. (cont.)

TERES, RHOMBOIDS, AND LATISSIMUS

Subject lies supine with knees bent up and both arms straight overhead, with upper arms close to ears. If arms lie flat on table overhead, upper back muscles are usually of normal length. If arms do not lie on table, then upper back muscles are short and require stretching.

Good stretches for a tight upper back are Numbers 1 and 3, from the *New Power Program* pp 52-53, the stretches shown in Figure 15 above, and those shown in Figure 16 on next page.

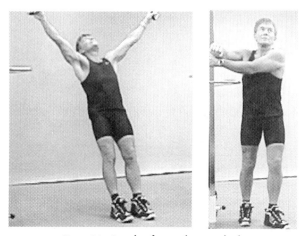

Figure 16. Stretches for a tight upper back.

HIP FLEXORS

Numerous muscles act to flex the hip. Major players are the one-joint iliopsoas, adductor longus, adductor brevis, two anterior sections of the adductor magnus and the pectineus, all of which cross only the hip joint. These work in conjunction with the two-joint muscles: the rectus femoris of the quadriceps, the tensor fascia lata, the sartorius, and the gracilis, all of which cross both hip and knee joints.

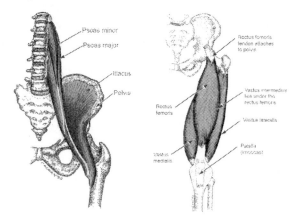

Figure 17. Major muscles that act to flex the hip. (Gluteus maximus, vastus medialis and vastus lateralis excepted).

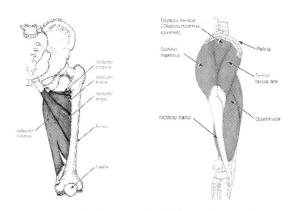

Figure 17. Major muscles that act to flex the hip. (Gluteus maximus, vastus medialis and vastus lateralis excepted). (cont.)

It is beyond the scope of this course to define restriction on hip flexion by individual muscles, but we will go part of the way and differentiate between one-joint and two-joint muscle tightness.

Subject lies supine on the table with knees hanging freely over one end. With hands behind thigh, subject pulls up one knee just sufficient for the back to lose its neutral lumbar curve and rest flat on the table. Buttock must remain on the table. In this position the pelvis is in posterior tilt by 5-10°.

If thigh of hanging leg remains in contact with the table, and knee of hanging leg flexes 70-90°, then hip flexors are usually of normal length.

If thigh leaves the table, but knee remains flexed 70-90°, then one-joint hip flexors are short.

If thigh remains on the table but knee flexes less than 70°, then two-joint hip flexors are short.

If thigh leaves the table and knee flexes less than 70°, then both one-joint and two-joint hip flexors are short.

STRETCHING HIP FLEXORS

Good stretches for tight one-joint hip flexors are Stretches 3 and 4 of The Vital Fifteen in the *New Power Program*, as shown in Figure 18. Good stretches for tight two-joint hip flexors are Stretches 5, 7, 8 and 14 of the Vital Fifteen as shown in Figure 19.

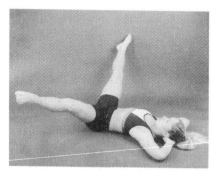
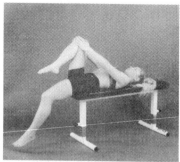

Figure 18. Stretches for tight one-joint hip flexors.

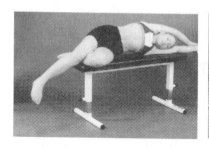
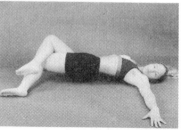
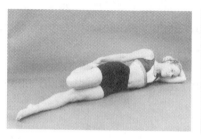
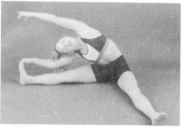

Figure 19. Stretches for tight two-joint hip flexors.

If subjects have short one-joint hip flexors, warn them to avoid any lunging stretches, such as Stretches 9 and 10 of The Vital Fifteen, as these will increase any excess lumbar curve. Especially warn all subjects with short hip flexors to avoid the common stretches, such as the hurdler, reverse hurdler, standing hamstring and others known to be harmful, shown on pp 42 and 43 of the *New Power Program.*

TENSOR FASCIA LATA

The tensor fascia lata deserves special mention, because of the common confusion of this muscle with the iliotibial band, which is its connecting tendon and should not be stretched. The tensor is easily tested for tightness using the old but reliable Obers Test.

Subject lies on table on side with head on bent arm, other arm relaxed in front, leg on table flexed at hip and knee, to stabilize pelvis front-to-back. Examiner stands behind subject with one hand on iliac crest, holding pelvis down firmly to keep it horizontally neutral and keep trunk on table. Trunk may not touch the table at the waist for some slim subjects.

Keeping uppermost thigh neutral (neither externally or internally rotated, abducted or adducted), move thigh back in extension with hand on shin. Release shin allowing thigh to drop into adduction. A drop of 10-20° indicates that the tensor is of normal length. Less than 10° indicates tensor tightness. More than 20° indicates excess tensor length.

Do not stretch already long tensors. For short tensors use the abductor stretch shown in Figure 19 (upper left).

HAMSTRINGS

The three major hamstrings are the semitendinosus, the semimembranosus and the long head of the biceps femoris. These are two-joint muscles, crossing both hip and knee joints, which flex the knee and extend the hip. For knee flexion they are assisted by the one-joint popliteus and the short head of the biceps femoris, both of which cross only the knee.

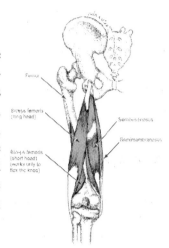

Figure 20. Hamstrings.

Subject lies supine with lumbar spine, sacrum, and legs flat on table. Subjects with short hip flexors will not be able to assume this position and will need a pad under the knees. That is why it is important to always test the hip flexors before the hamstrings. Otherwise, short hip flexors will cause normal length hamstrings to appear short. Examiner holds one thigh down firmly, then raises the other leg straight, with the knee fully extended but the foot relaxed to limit gastrocnemius involvement.

With normal length hamstrings, the angle between the legs reaches 80-90° before the knee starts to flex. If the angle exceeds 90°, the hamstrings are too long and should not be stretched further in any exercise program, for risk of making the knee and hip joints unstable.

If the angle is less than 80°, the hamstrings are short and require stretching. The best stretches are Number 6 of The Vital 15, assisted by Number 1 for the piriformis and other small muscles of the pelvis. These are shown in Figure 21.

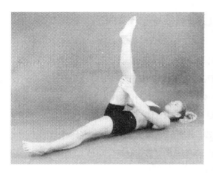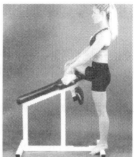

Figure 21. Stretches for tight hamstrings.

Do not attempt to test hamstrings using the old bending-to-touch-toes nonsense, as it inextricably combines five different sets of muscles and connective tissues, the three curves of the back, the hamstrings, and the gastrocnemius. The same goes for the seated-bending-forward-to-touch-the-toes, even though you see countless commercial devices in gyms everywhere that carry on such codswallop.

As Kendall documents,[12] subjects can pass or fail these tests because of abnormal flexion of the spine, **or** abnormal length of hamstrings, **or** abnormal length of gastrocnemius, **or** because of individual variations in arm length, **or** because of individual variations in leg length. So what the hell are you measuring? Along with the senseless how-many-pushups-you-can-do-in-a-minute, these tests were developed as a quick and nasty way to screen recruits for the First World War – and that's where they should have stayed!

MUSCLES OF THE CORE

We have already covered the major support, rotation, and extensor muscles of the back that form part of the core: the iliocostalis, longissimus, quadratus lumborum, and serratus posterior inferior. Now we will look at the lateral flexors and rotators of the trunk (internal and external obliques), and support and flexor muscles of the trunk (transversus and abdominus rectus). All are shown below.

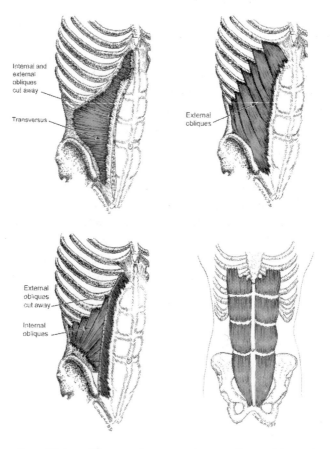

Figure 22. Lateral flexors and rotators and anterior flexors of the trunk.

TESTING ABDOMINAL STRENGTH

Abdominal strength in flexing the trunk is commonly divided into upper and lower abdominals of the abdominus rectus. Upper abdominals are commonly tested by the supine-trunk-curl-sit-up, and lower abdominals by the supine-straight-leg-lowering-with-flat-back.[12] Solemnly following such flapdoodle makes trainers look clever, but measures nothing of value. Still, it does help keep them out of real sports training where they are likely to do a lot of damage.

Basic physiology shows clearly that the eight heads of the abdominus rectus act all of a piece, and that they cannot work without also involving the internal and external obliques and the transversus, even though several different nerves are involved.[13] You can devise movements that put the top heads of the rectus under a bit more strain than the bottom heads, but they are of little use in determining basic core strength, because the stronger heads and the other muscles will always take over the movement as exhaustion occurs.

All sit-up movements from the floor also involve a degree of hip flexion, even with the back flat, and whether the legs are straight or bent. The abdominals do not cross the hip joint, so hip flexors are always involved too. All leg-lowering tests also involve a lot of hip flexor action in eccentric contraction. And leg raising – forget it! It's mainly hip flexion all the way.

The widespread misuse of these tests has hurt a lot of athletes. We have measured many Olympic athletes with cores of steel, that fail the leg lowering test miserably, because they have a huge gluteus maximus. Their big strong butts lever the lumbar spine off the floor long before their legs get near it. Then there are the folk with short hip flexors. Their pelvises get yanked into anterior tilt, and the spine leaves the floor, by the time their legs are half-way down. The leg lowering test is useful only in the hands of medical experts, and then only for measuring the gross weaknesses in the frail and sedentary patients it was designed for.

In real life movements, hip flexion and abdominal flexion are inextricably intertwined, and that's the way they should be measured in any exercise program that purports to produce a stronger, more functional body.

The basic tests we use are done hanging from a bar. First is the Knee Kicks. Minimal acceptable abdominal/ hip flexor strength in males, is the ability to kick the knees up to the upper chest from straight down just forward of the pelvis, while curling the trunk, for eight repetitions. In females the figure is five repetitions.

Basic abdominal/hip flexor strength for athletes, both male and female, is the ability to raise straight legs from a dead hang to touch the bar once between the hands. A really strong athlete can do 30 repetitions. These tests from the *New Power Program*, which are also used as remedial exercises, are shown in Figure 23.

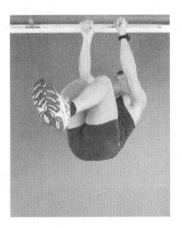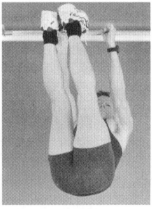

Figure 23. Basic tests for abdominals/hip flexor strength.

PRESCRIPTION FOR A TOP TRAINER

This brief introduction to postural and structural analysis forms part of the Posture and Flexibility Section of the Certification for Trainers in the Colgan Power Program. It is the essential first step to designing effective resistance programs both for athletes and for the general public. In summary, designing a full program proceeds in the following nine steps.

1. Analyse posture and structure.

2. Test for muscle length.

3. Test for muscle strength.

4. Use this text plus The Colgan *Power Program* and Lee Parore's *Power Posture* to design remedial exercises to:
   a. Correct postural defects.
   b. Stretch the tight muscles
   c. Strengthen the weak muscles.

5. Design an individual Extension/Connection Cycle from the Colgan Power Program to strengthen connective tissues.

6. Design an individual Strength/Stabilization Cycle from the Colgan Power Program to strengthen prime movers and stabilizers simultaneously.

7. Design an individual Power Cycle from the Colgan Power Program to integrate the previous cycles into a single unit of powerful movement.

8. Design an individual Link Cycle from the Colgan Power Program, matched to the subject's sport and performance goals, to train the nervous system for speed.

9. In the second year, design an individual Coordination Cycle from the Advanced Colgan Power Program to improve balance, agility, coordination, and fluidity of movement.

FORM 1
FOR POSTURAL AND STRUCTURAL ANALYSIS.

Name: _____

Date: _____

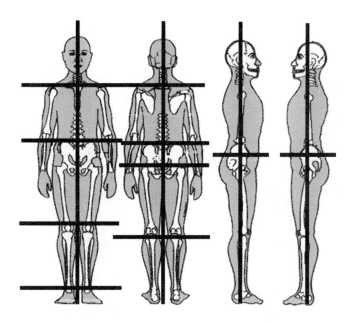

FORM 2
FOR POSTURAL AND STRUCTURAL ANALYSIS.

Name: _____

Date: _____

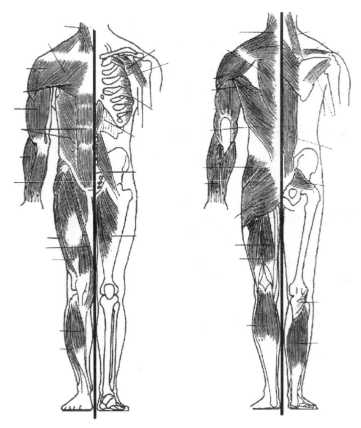

Muscles most in need of stretching.

FORM 3
FOR POSTURAL AND STRUCTURAL ANALYSIS.

Name: _____

Date: _____

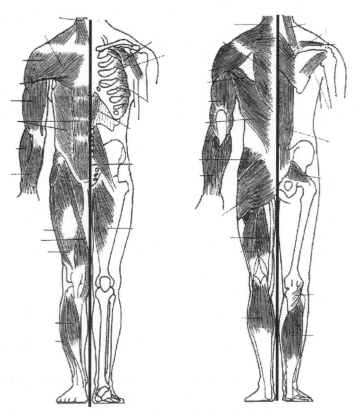

Muscles most in need of strengthening.

REFERENCES

1. Centers for Disease Control. **Morbidity and Mortality Weekly Report,** 1989;38:449-453.
2. Centers for Disease Control. **Morbidity and Mortality Weekly Report.** 1992;24 January:33-35.
3. Brownson RC et al. Measuring physical activity with the behavioral risk factor surveillance system. **Med Sci Sports Exerc.** 2000;32:1913-1918.
4. Centers for Disease Control. **Morbidity and Mortality Weekly Report.** 2001;50:758-761.
5. Chakravarthy MV et al. An obligation for primary care physicians to prescribe physical activity to sedentary patients to reducw the risk of chronic health conditions. **Mayo Clinic Proc.** 2002;77:165-173.
6. Thompson LV. Skeletal muscle adaptations with age, inactivity, and therapeutic exercise. **Orthop Sports Phys Ther**. 2002;32:44-57.
7. Inman VT. Human locomotion. **Can Med Assoc J.** 1996;94:1047-1054.
8. Colgan M. **The New Power Program**. Vancouver: Apple Publishing 2001.
9. Travell J. **Myofascial Dysfunction and Pain, Second Edition. Volume 1.** Baltimore: Williams and Wilkins, 1999.
10. Minimo AM, Smith BL. Deaths: Preliminary data for 2000. **Natl Vital Stat Rep.** 2001;49:1-40.
11. Basmajian JV, Deluca CJ. **Muscles Alive, Fifth Edition**. Baltimore:Williams and Wilkins. 1985.
12. Kendall FP et al. **Muscle Testing and Function, Fourth Edition,** Baltimore: Williams and Wilkins, 1993.
13. Travell J **Myofascial Dysfunction and Pain, Second Edition, Volume 2.** Baltimore: Williams and Wilkins, 1999.
14. Parore L. **Power Posture.** Vancouver: Apple Publishing, 2002.